Alkaline Smoothies

Alkaline Smoothie Recipes for Weight Loss
and the Benefits of an Alkaline Diet - Alkaline
Drinks Your Way to Vibrant Health - Massive
Energy and Natural Weight Loss

Sheldon Miller

ISBN-13: 978-1722213992

ISBN-10: 172221399X

Table of Content

Introduction

Scientifically speaking, it is often believed that the most effective and efficient diet programs are the ones that work with the body's natural internal mechanism and systems and aids them in improving the overall health.

That being said, amongst the plethora of similar diets out there in the market right now, it seems that no other food can fend off diseases and improve mortality rate other than the incredible Alkaline diet!

The core concept behind the Alkaline diet is pretty simple, which makes it even more accessible and more comfortable to follow than other complicated programs out there.

To summarize, the diet requires an individual to cut down on processed junk food and unhealthy habits that induce acidosis and to replace them with a variety of Alkaline ingredients (that mostly includes fresh fruits and vegetables!).

Asides from vastly improving your health in the long run, correctly following the regime will:

- Aid in weight loss
- Help increase your overall health
- Strengthen your immune system
- Increase the amount of energy available to your body

Sounds interesting right?

But wait! You must wonder, "How I can ever hope to follow this diet while having such a hectic lifestyle of my own?"

Well, Smoothies are the solution to that problem!

These are easy to make and take the extremely minimal amount of time and effort, but the payout is huge!

The body readily absorbs smoothies, and you will be able to reap the benefits of your Alkaline Regime in no time!

I have tried my very best to make this book as accessible and easy to understand as possible! In doing so, I have included two pretty detailed intro chapters covering the basics of the Alkaline Diet and Alkaline Smoothies.

This is followed by loads of amazing Alkaline Smoothie recipes that you are sure to enjoy!

I bid you a happy and healthy life!

Chapter 1: The Core Concept Of Going Alkaline

Despite being a pretty popular form of diet these days, the core concepts of Alkaline Diet are still widely misunderstood by a lot of people! Especially the ones who are newly trying to break into this fantastic program!

But due to the lack of having a good understanding of the fundamental of Alkalinity in our body, people often tend to completely ignore the necessity to maintain a proper pH, which ultimately leads to various diseases in the long run.

If you happen to be one of those former individuals, then I would highly recommend that you go through this chapter to get a good understanding of the core concepts of Alkaline Diet.

This will help you not only to understand better how the Smoothies will help your body but also inspire you to shift from Smoothies and follow a full-fledged Alkaline Diet for a healthy future!

That being said, we must begin with the core concept first.

The Core Idea of Going Alkaline

So, the fundamental principle that governs the idea of following an Alkaline program is pretty straightforward actually and is based on a straightforward philosophy that tells us that:

"The internal chemistry of our body is large altered depending on the type of food that we consume."

To use more specific terms, the "pH" value of our body drastically changes depending on the type of food that we eat and determines whether the internal condition is acidic or alkaline. Initially, these terms might seem a little confusing to you, but don't worry as I will explain them in the coming pages.

Right now though, let me talk a little bit more about the way the internal condition changes. But before moving forward, you must learn to appreciate the fact that whenever our body requires energy, it starts to burn down food. The whole process of breaking down foods into tiny molecules takes place inside the cells in a very well-balanced and strictly maintained internal environment.

Once the food is broken down into its elementary compounds and the energy is absorbed, it tends to leave behind a form of residue that is known as "Ash" in scientific terms. This "Ash" is ultimately responsible for determining whether the consumed food is acidic, alkaline or neutral. Consequently, these ashes are responsible for the changes in pH level in our body.

The bottom line here is that if your body is exposed to a higher amount of acidic "Ash," it slowly starts to become more vulnerable to diseases as the immune system weakens.

Alternatively, when your body experiences a high level of Alkalinity in the bloodstream, an extra layer of protection starts to form that seems to impact the health of our body positively.

And to explain the different types of Ashes further, we have:

- **Acidic:** Produce such as meat, fish, poultry, dairy, grains, eggs and even alcohol are considered to be acidic.
- **Neutral:** Foods such as sugars, fats or starches are said to be neutral
- **Alkaline:** Foods including vegetables, legume, nuts, and Fruits are said to be Alkaline.

The main aim of the Alkaline diet is to encourage your body into eating/drinking food that is more Alkaline to slightly increase the pH and create a more alkaline internal environment.

Eating more Alkaline food also helps to tackle the adverse effects of acidosis and prevents the body from going into an Acidic state entirely.

As a general rule of thumb, the pH level of 7.4 is regarded as optimal for human beings (which is slightly Alkaline).

The diet tries to maintain and balance this pH to improve health quality.

The huge amount of benefits is discussed in details in the second chapter.

Understanding pH

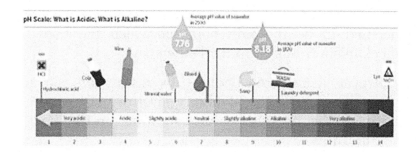

pH Scale: What is Acidic, What is Alkaline?

Now that you have a good grasp of the core concept of Alkaline diet let me explain the concept of "pH" levels.

A good understanding of pH levels is exceptionally crucial to comprehend further how Alkaline diet works.

So, generally speaking, pH is a component of our blood that is known as the "Potential of Hydrogen."

While assessing the level of pH in liquid, it is possible to determine whether a liquid is alkaline, acidic or neutral.

Regarding humans, we usually measure the acidity or alkalinity of body fluids and tissue.

The measurement is done on a scale of 0-14 (refer to the picture above). The standard convention of reading the scale is as follows:

- The lower the pH value, the more acidic a solution is
- The higher the value goes, the more alkaline the solution is

- 7 is considered to be the neutral point on the scale

The pH level of our body usually stays at 7.4, which is deemed to be the safe point at which the body's mechanism works at optimal efficiency.

However, it has been deduced by researchers that a slight increase in the alkalinity level of pH tends to improve the overall health condition of the body significantly.

It should be noted though that the pH level of the body varies from one region to the next. For example, the stomach is generally regarded as naturally being the most acidic part of the body.

If the natural level of pH gets altered by even a slight amount, the body of human beings, as well as many other organisms, starts to react negatively.

A good example would be the recent increase of Carbon Di-Oxide disposition which led to a substantial a slight decrease in the ocean's pH, where it went to 8.1 from 8.2. And a 0.1 change in pH, means various aquatic organism and life forms have started to suffer.

This pH level is not only essential for plant growth but also forms part of the minerals in our food.

But every single organism has several means of defending the body from such changes. In the case of human beings, various minerals contribute by acting as a "buffer" to normalize the pH level of our body should it become more acidic!

Understanding the Two Extremes, Acidosis and Alkalosis

Maintaining your pH is exceptionally crucial as even very subtle changes in your body pH can bring about drastic results!

Depending on your pH level, your body can experience one of the two extremes.

If the pH increases a lot, then your body will become too alkaline and experience "Alkalosis."

On the hand, if your body pH level lowers down to a higher degree, it starts to experience Acidosis.

During Alkalosis, you will start to experience loss of electrolytes, lower oxygen levels and suffer from various organ malfunctions.

Symptoms of Alkalosis includes

- Confusion
- Lightheadedness
- Twitching
- Sudden muscle spasm
- Seizure
- Respiratory problems
- Tingling in facial extremities

Alternatively, when the pH of your body drops too much, it becomes acidic, and your body experiences "Acidosis."

During this state, you will experience the following symptoms:

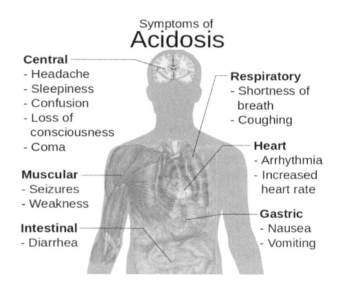

- Metabolic problems
- Respiratory problems
- Lactic imbalance
- Renal complications
- Increased risk of cardiovascular diseases
- Diabetes
- Insulin Resistance
- Kidney Damage
- Confusion
- Fatigue
- Breathlessness
- Lethargy

A much more worrying matter is the fact that without a proper food program, you can very quickly push your body into a state of Acidosis!

But, to prevent that from happening, your body does come equipped with its natural mechanism.

How the Body Defends Itself

Our body is very well equipped when it comes to naturally defending itself from various diseases and health issues.

The natural feedback system also allows the body to keep itself protected from sudden changes in pH! Thanks to the fantastic job of our Kidneys, we are kept safe from the harmful effects of Acidosis.

How?

Well, whenever the acid level of our body tends to increase, the Kidney starts to send the excess acid to the bladder, which is later on excreted through urination.

The Kidney also helps to maintain the levels of bicarbonate in our body that helps to tackle unwanted acidic effects as well.

However, that's not to say that the kidney can save the day all the time!

In worst case scenarios where the Acidic level goes beyond the tolerable capacity of the kidney, health complications begin to show up.

Early on, these complications won't be dangerous; however, they will increase with time.

You should be aware though that the kidneys aren't the only organ that helps to maintain a proper pH level!

In fact, the lungs play a significant role too.

Carbon Di Oxide is the by-product of cellular metabolism, but the problem occurs if it starts to get mixed with the blood as it causes it to become acidic.

The lungs help to get rid of CO_2 from the body and thus maintain an excellent acid-alkaline balance in our body.

The dietary list that you will need to know and follow during your Smoothie journey is provided in the next chapter. However, there are certain habits that you should try to refrain yourself from to maximize the efficiency of the program.

Habits to avoid

- Refrain yourself from the usage of drugs or alcohol
- Prevent yourself from consuming large quantities of caffeine
- Prevent yourself from using a large number of antibiotics
- Try to avoid artificial sweeteners
- Try to keep yourself free from chronic stress
- Try to maintain a proper fiber intake
- Avoid doing exercises
- Going for excess animal meat mostly from inorganic sources
- Ingestion of hormones through artificial means such as medicines or beauty products
- Exposing our body to radiation from cleaners, computers, microwaves, cell phones
- Using preservatives or any form of food coloring
- Getting exposed to herbicides or pesticides

- Extreme cases of pollution
- Eating refined or "processed" foods
- Breathing shallowly

That pretty much covers the basics of the Alkaline concept, in the next chapter we will talk a little bit about the benefits of Alkaline Smoothies!

Chapter 2: Why Alkaline Smoothies?

It has been scientifically proven that the best and effective diets are mostly the ones that work with the body's natural process and internal environment to bring about positive changes.

As you can already tell, the Alkaline diet is one such program that does not require any artificial external stimulus to work!

Instead, the health benefits from this diet can be reaped solely by consuming 100% natural and healthy ingredients.

Now, I understand that with such a hectic and busy lifestyle, it is often challenging to manage enough time to prepare a hearty homemade meal! But making a Smoothie? It takes only 5-10 minutes, but the health benefits are abundant!

Speaking of health benefits:

Surprising Benefits of Alkaline Smoothie Diet Are

- **Greatly aids in protecting the muscle density and bone mass of the body:** The primary route through which alkaline smoothies can do this is by balancing out the ratio of the essential elements that are required for muscle and bone development. These include magnesium, calcium, and phosphate. Alkaline Diet also encourages the growth of Vitamin D absorption and development of growth hormones which further helps to amplify the strength of the bones. Also, it assist the body in tackling some variety chronic diseases.

- **Dramatically lowers down the risk of stroke and hypertension:** One of the more potent effects of an Alkaline Smoothies is that it greatly helps to lower down the inflammation caused due to an increase in the levels of growth hormones. There have been proven cases where alkaline smoothies has been shown to improve the overall cardiovascular health of the body, wherein the body learns to protect itself from various problems such as high cholesterol build up, kidney stone formation, stroke, hypertension and even memory loss.

- **Dramatically lowers down Chronic Pain and inflammation:** Multiple studies have shown that there is a secure connection between a perfectly balanced Alkaline diet/Alkaline Smoothie Diet and a decreased level of Chronic Pain. It has been studied and found that Chronic Acidosis significantly contributes to problems such as muscle spasms, chronic back pain, menstrual symptoms, headaches, joint pain, and inflammation. Regular exposure to Alkaline content will lower or reduce Acidosis, thus mitigating the harmfulness of these symptoms.

- **Considerably helps to enhance the absorption of Vitamin and lower Magnesium Deficiency:** Magnesium is required for the proper functioning for at least a hundred different enzymes found in our body. Most people who have suffered from magnesium deficiency have complained that they have experienced significant heart problems, symptoms of insomnia, muscle aches, headaches and also chronic anxiety. Since alkaline diet radically helps to increase the overall Magnesium of the body, it helps to mitigate all of these effects. And as a bonus, it also helps to prevent Vitamin D deficiency which further increases the strength of the immune system and the functioning of the endocrine system.

- **Helps to improve the overall immune functions of the body while protecting it from Cancer:** When the cells of the body are deprived of minerals that are required to dispose the waste of the body properly or to provide the body with the required oxygen, the overall biological architecture of the body starts to suffer altogether significantly. The minerals loss dramatically affects the absorption of Vitamins while at the same time the pathogens and toxins begin to gather around the body in this weakened state.

Various researchers established in the British Journal of Radiology have shown that the process through which cancerous cells are killed (apoptosis) occurs in a more considerable percentage in a body which has an overall Alkaline internal environment.

- **Aids in weight loss:** Since in Alkaline Smoothie Diet, you are restricting yourself from the consumption of acid-forming foods and are opting for more alkaline inducing foods. Consequently, you are preparing your body to prevent itself from obesity by lowering down the levels of inflammation and Leptin in your body. Both of these contribute to the reducing hunger while enhancing the fat burning capabilities of our body.

Since the foods that are suited for Alkaline Diet are also the very same foods that are high in Anti-Inflammatory properties! Consuming them helps your body to considerably maintain a reasonable level Leptin level that, in turn, allows the body to feel full after eating just a small amount of calories.

- **Appreciably increase the available energy of the body:** The pH level of our body hugely affects our cell's ability to produce and process ATP (Adenosine Triphosphate) which is the chemical that supplies our body with energy. If the internal conditions of our body start to get too acidic, then ATP production won't take place correctly, and soon you will begin to feel lethargic from time to time. This can very easily be prevented by the consumption of Alkaline Foods to maintain a higher PH.

- **Improve the health of your Teeth and Gum:** If the acid levels around your mouth get too high, it creates an optimum environment for bacteria to grow at a more accelerated rate. These bacteria can result in some different complications, including bad breath and gum disease, thus leading to tooth decay. Providing a more Alkaline condition here will much help the body to lessen the likelihood of such things happening.

- **Slow down the process of aging:** Whenever the cells of our body are exposed to a highly acidic environment, they start to lose their proper functionalities. This dramatically prevents the cells from repairing themselves properly, which, in turn, results in accelerated aging. Again, this can be avoided by going on an Alkaline Diet as well.

- **Enhanced Sexual Drive:** After a great deal of research, it has been scientifically proven that acidic conditions in our body lead to decreases sexual performance. This can be avoided by going for foods that are Alkaline as an internal

Alkaline Condition will significantly help to enhance your sexual performance as well.

And those are the just the tip of the Ice-Berg! There are a whole lot more where that came from.

What to have and what not to have

When deciding to create your Smoothie, it is best if you can stick to the following ingredients as closely as possible for maximum benefits:

- Mushroom
- Citrus
- Dates
- Raisins
- Spinach
- Grapefruit
- Tomatoes
- Avocados
- Summer Black Radish
- Alfalfa Grass
- Barley Grass
- Oregano
- Cucumber
- Kale
- Jicama
- Wheat Grass
- Broccoli
- Garlic
- Ginger
- Green Beans
- Endive

- Cabbage
- Celery
- Red Beet
- Watermelon
- Figs
- Ripe Bananas
- Almonds
- Navy beans
- Lima Beans
- Coconut milk
- Almond Milk
- Greek Yogurt

Alternatively, the following ingredients are strictly prohibited if you want to maintain your Alkaline streak properly!

Let me elaborate on the foods first. So, in general, you should try to avoid

- Processed foods that are high in sodium as they significantly cause the blood vessels of becoming constricted and results in acidity
- Conventional meats or Cold Cut Meats
- Processed Cereals such as Chocos or Corn Flakes
- Eggs
- Lentils
- Alcohol and Caffeinated Beverages
- Produces made of grain, regardless of being "Whole' grain or not.
- Products that are extremely rich in Calcium can lead to severe cases of Osteoporosis!
- Walnuts and Peanuts

- Rice, Pasta or any other package products made of "Grain."

And with that, you are now fully equipped with all the information required to embark on your Smoothie Journey.

But just as a bonus and to make the book complete, let me share a little bit information regarding Smoothie making as well.

The secret "six" steps to perfect Smoothie

If you want, you can follow the steps outlined in the recipes of this book! In fact, most of the recipes in this book follow the outline that I will discuss here.

However, it is always better to know the Science or the underlying technology behind everything right?

Just like an excellent solution to a problem. Smoothies also have a formula that acts as the hidden "Key" to creating the perfect Smoothie.

It is as follows:

> **Choose Smoothie Recipe + Add Liquid + Add Base + Add Fruits/Veggies + Add Optional Mix-Ins + Blend= Ground Breaking Smoothie Ready!**

Let me break down the components individually for you.

The Recipe

The recipe will always act as the foundation of the Smoothie that you are making. In our case, since we are trying to balance out acidic contents, always try to look for recipes that include Alkaline ingredients in its list.

The Liquid

Once you have decided your recipe, the next step is to start adding the contents to your blender. A prudent decision is first to add the liquid ingredients.

Follow the recipe and look for the liquids in the ingredients list, add them one by one.

In case you are experimenting, good options for liquid include:

- Almond milk
- Coconut milk
- Organic fruit juice (fresh)
- Fresh/squeeze juice
- Tea

The Base

The "base" is what is responsible for giving your Smoothie the interesting creamy texture. You may think of the base as the "Body" of the smoothie.

Good examples for the base include:

- Bananas
- Mango
- Peach
- Pear
- Apple
- Avocado

The Fruit/Veggies

Once you have added your base, now it's time to add your desired fruit and vegetable. This is pretty straightforward and follows the recipe accordingly. However, good options to experiment with include:

- Spinach
- Kale
- Beet Greens
- Berries
- Lettuce
- Arugula
- Dandelion Greens

Etc.

Optional Mix-Ins

The final step is to add a little bit extra to fortify the texture of your Smoothie and significantly enhance its flavor.

Mix–ins may include:

- Salt
- Spices
- Protein Powder
- Superfoods

Once you are done adding all the ingredients, blend it up and enjoy! Depending on your ingredients, it's best to start off with low settings during blending and to climb up to higher settings of the food processor eventually.

Common Smoothie Blunders

If you are an amateur Smoothie artist, then it is very natural that you may face some difficulties early on. The following tips should help you deal with some of the most common issues:

- **Too Frothy:** If frothiness is the issue, try to add a little less liquid and not blend it for too long. Alternatively, you may withhold a portion of the liquid and gradually added it later on once the other half of the ingredients are properly blended. Keep in mind that when using base ingredients such as Avocado, banana, etc. you won't need much liquid as they already have a fair amount of liquid on their own.

- **Too Runny:** If you find your Smoothie to be too runny, lower down the amount of liquid and add more thickening ingredients.

- **Not sweet enough/tasty:** Add a bit of your desired natural sweetener, honey, dates or maple syrup are good options.

- **Too bitter:** An excellent way to tackle bitterness is to lower the number of greens and add some fruits.

- **Not blending correctly:** If you find that you are unable to blend your ingredients properly, try to cut them into small pieces and add them to your blender. This usually solves the problem.

Chapter 3: The Smoothies Galore

Hearty Alkaline Strawberry Summer Deluxe

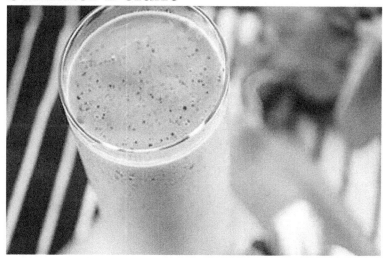

Serving: 2

Prep Time: 5 minutes

<u>Ingredients</u>

- ½ cup organic strawberries/blueberries
- Half of a banana
- 2 cups coconut water
- ½ inch ginger
- Juice of 2 grapefruits

Cooking Directions

1. Add all the listed ingredients to your blender
2. Blend until smooth
3. Add a few ice cubes and serve the smoothie
4. Enjoy!

Delish Pineapple and Coconut Milk Smoothie

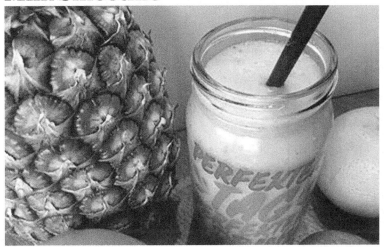

Serving: 2

Prep Time: 5 minutes

Ingredients

- ¼ cup pineapple, frozen
- ¾ cup coconut milk

Cooking Directions

1. Add the listed ingredients to your blender and blend well with settings on high
2. Once the mixture is smooth, pour smoothie in a tall glass and serve
3. Chill and enjoy!

The Minty Refresher

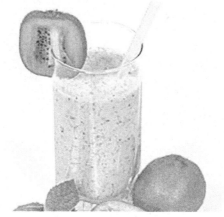

Serving: 2

Prep Time: 5 minutes

Ingredients

- 2 cups mint tea
- 1 cucumber, peeled
- 2 green apples
- 1 cup blueberries
- Stevia (to sweeten)
- Few slices of lime/lemon for garnish

Cooking Directions

1. Add the listed ingredients to your blender and blend until smooth
2. Add ice and sweeten with a bit of stevia
3. Garnish with lime/lemon slices
4. Serve and enjoy!

The "Upbeat" Strawberry and Clementine Glass

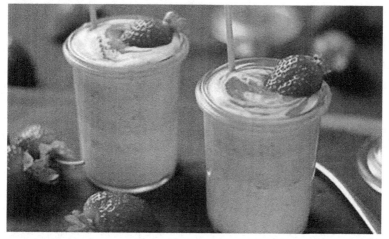

Serving: 2

Prep Time: 5 minutes

Ingredients

- 8 ounces strawberries, fresh
- 1 banana, chopped into chunks
- 2 Clementines / Mandarins

Cooking Directions

1. Peel the Clementines and remove seeds
2. Add the listed ingredients to your blender/food processor and blend until smooth
3. Serve chilled and enjoy!

Cabbage and Coconut Chia Smoothie

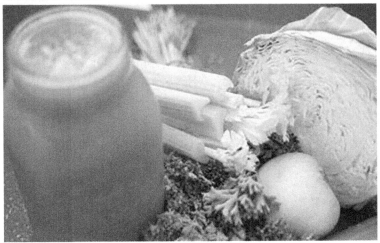

Serving: 2

Prep Time: 5 minutes

Ingredients

- 1/3 cup cabbage
- 1 cup cold unsweetened coconut milk
- 1 tablespoon chia seeds
- ½ cup cherries
- ½ cup spinach

Cooking Directions

1. Add coconut milk to your blender
2. Cut cabbage and add to your blender
3. Place chia seeds in a coffee grinder and chop to powder, brush the powder into your blender
4. Pit the cherries and add them to your blender

5. Wash and dry the spinach and chop
6. Add to the mix
7. Cover and blend on low followed by medium
8. Taste the texture and serve chilled!

The Cherry Beet Delight

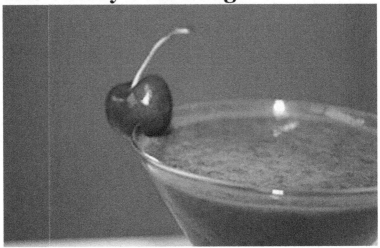

Serving: 2

Prep Time: 5 minutes

Ingredients

- 1 cup cherries, pitted
- ½ cup beets
- Few banana slices
- 1 cup water, filtered, alkaline
- 1 cup coconut milk
- Pinch of organic vanilla powder
- Pinch of cinnamon
- Pinch of stevia
- Few mint leaves/lime slices to garnish

Cooking Directions

1. Add berries, beets, water, banana slices, coconut milk to your blender

2. Blend well until smooth
3. Add more water if the texture is too creamy for you
4. Add coconut oil, vanilla, cinnamon, and stir
5. Add a bit of stevia for extra sweetness
6. Garnish with mint leaves and lime slices
7. Enjoy!

The Avocado Paradise

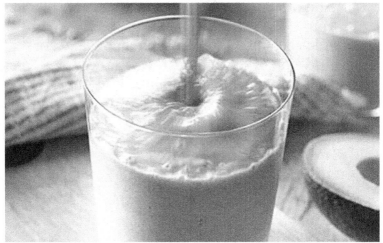

Serving: 2

Prep Time: 5 minutes

Ingredients

- ½ avocado, cubed
- 1 cup coconut milk
- Half a lemon
- ¼ cup fresh spinach leaves
- 1 pear
- 1 tablespoon hemp. Seed powder

Toppings

- Handful of macadamia nuts
- Handful of grapes
- 2 lemon slices

Cooking Directions

1. Blend all the ingredients until smooth
2. Add a few ice cubes to make it chilled
3. Add your desired toppings
4. Enjoy!

The Authentic Vegetable Medley

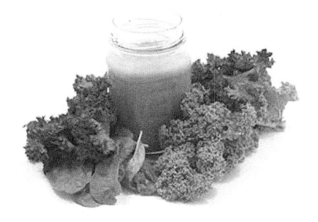

Serving: 2

Prep Time: 5 minutes

Ingredients

- 1 cup broccoli, steamed
- 1 bunch asparagus, steamed
- 2 cups coconut milk
- 2 tablespoons coconut oil
- 2 carrots, peeled
- Few inch horseradish
- Himalayan salt
- Pinch of chili powder
- ½ a onion
- 2 garlic cloves

Cooking Directions

1. Add all the listed ingredients to your blender except coconut oil, salt and chili powder
2. Blend until smooth
3. Add salt, coconut oil, and chili powder
4. Stir well, and serve chilled!

The Original Power Producer

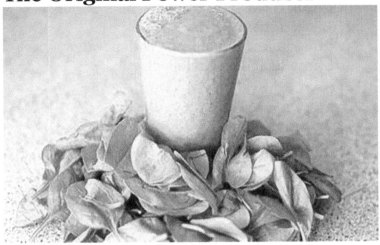

Serving: 2

Prep Time: 5 minutes

Ingredients

- ½ cup spinach
- 1 avocado, diced
- 1 cup coconut milk
- 1 tablespoon flax seed
- 2 nori sheets, roasted and crushed
- 1 garlic clove
- Salt to taste

Toppings

- Handful of pistachios
- 3 tablespoons bell pepper, finely chopped
- A handful of parsley leaves

Cooking Directions

1. Blend all the ingredients until smooth
2. Add a few ice cubes to make it chilled
3. Add your desired toppings
4. Enjoy!

The Dreamy Cherry Mix

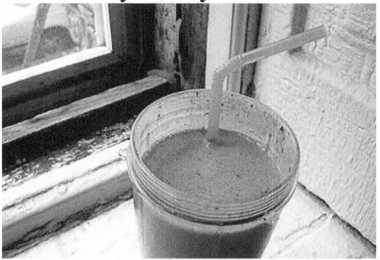

Serving: 2

Prep Time: 5 minutes

Ingredients

- ½ cup ripe cherries
- Juice of 1 lemon
- 1 cup coconut milk
- 1 avocado, cubed
- ¼ cup spinach
- Few slices of cucumber, peeled

Toppings

- Handful of pistachios
- Handful of raisins
- 1 slice lemon

Cooking Directions

1. Blend all the ingredients until smooth
2. Add a few ice cubes to make it chilled
3. Add your desired toppings
4. Enjoy!

Better Than Your Favorite Restaurant "Lemon Smoothie"

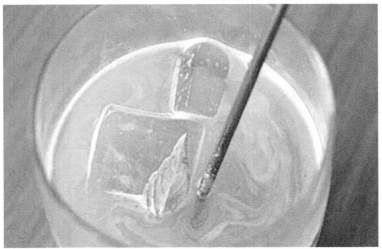

Serving: 2

Prep Time: 5 minutes

<u>Ingredients</u>

- 2 cups organic rice milk, gluten free
- 1 cup melon, chopped
- ½ an avocado, cubed
- ½ a cucumber, peeled and sliced
- Ice cubes
- 2 limes, juiced
- 1 tablespoon coconut oil
- Few banana slices to taste

Cooking Directions

1. Add the listed ingredients to your blender (except coconut oil) and blend well
2. Blend until you have a smooth texture
3. Add coconut oil and stir
4. Enjoy!

The "One" With the Watermelon

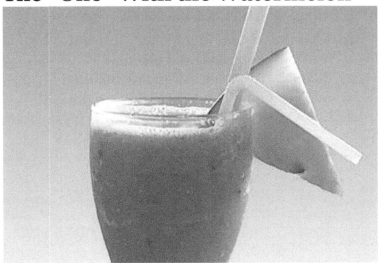

Serving: 2

Prep Time: 5 minutes

Ingredients

- 1 cup watermelon, sliced
- ½ cup coconut, shredded
- 1 grapefruit, cubed
- ½ cup coconut milk
- 2 tablespoons almond butter

Toppings

- Handful of crushed almonds
- Handful of raisins
- 2 tablespoons coconut powder

Cooking Directions

1. Blend all the ingredients until smooth
2. Add a few ice cubes to make it chilled
3. Add your desired toppings
4. Enjoy!

The Sweet Potato Acid Buster

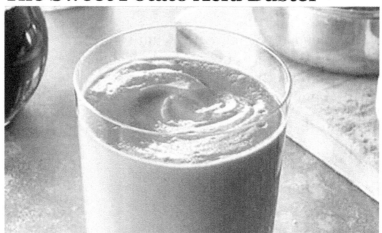

Serving: 2

Prep Time: 5 minutes

Ingredients

- 1 cup sweet potato, chopped
- 1 cup almond milk
- ¼ teaspoon nutmeg
- ¼ teaspoon ground cinnamon
- 1 teaspoon flax seed
- 1 small avocado, cubed
- Few spinach leaves, torn

Toppings

- Handful of crushed almonds
- Handful of crushed cashews
- 3 tablespoons orange juice

Cooking Directions

1. Blend all the ingredients until smooth
2. Add a few ice cubes to make it chilled
3. Add your desired toppings
4. Enjoy!

The Sunshine Offering

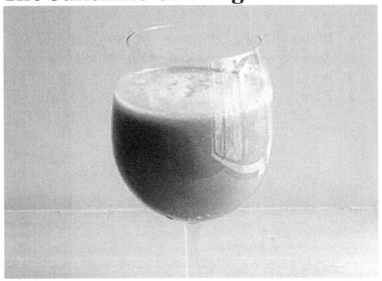

Serving: 2

Prep Time: 5 minutes

Ingredients

- 2 cups fresh spinach
- 1 and ½ cups almond milk
- ½ cup coconut water
- 3 cups fresh pineapple
- 2 tablespoons coconut unsweetened flakes

Cooking Directions

1. Add all the listed ingredients to your blender
2. Blend until smooth
3. Add a few ice cubes and serve the smoothie
4. Enjoy!

The Sleepy Bug Smoothie

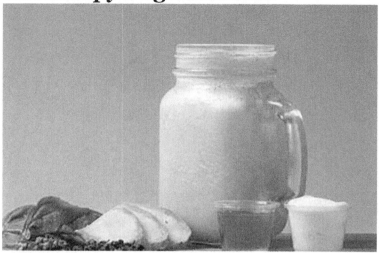

Serving: 2

Prep Time: 5 minutes

Ingredients

- 1 cup fennel tea infusion
- 1 cup almond milk
- 1 cup watermelon, chopped
- 1 green apple
- ½ cup pomegranate
- ½ inch ginger
- Stevia to sweeten

Cooking Directions

1. Add the listed ingredients to your blender
2. Blend until smooth
3. Add a bit of stevia if you want more sweetness
4. Serve chilled and enjoy!

Matcha Coconut Smoothie

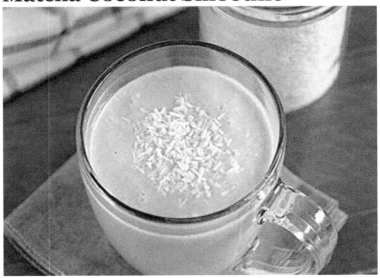

Serving: 2

Prep Time: 5 minutes

Ingredients

- 1 whole banana, cubed
- 1 cup frozen mango, chunked
- 2 kale leaves, torn
- 3 tablespoon white beans
- 2 tablespoon shredded coconut
- ½ teaspoon matcha green tea powder
- 1 cup water

How To

1. Add banana, kale, mango, matcha powder and white beans to your blender

2. Blend until you have a nice smoothie
3. Add shredded coconut as topping
4. Serve and enjoy!

Ravishing Apple and Cucumber Glass

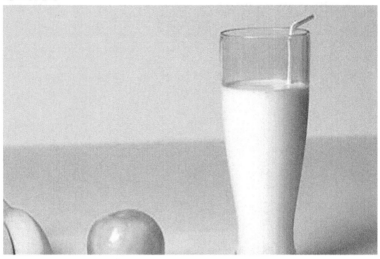

Serving: 2

Prep Time: 5 minutes

Ingredients

- 1 green apple
- 2 cucumbers, peeled
- 1 cup almond milk
- ½ cup coconut cream (raw and organic)
- Pinch of cinnamon and nutmeg (each)
- Pinch of Himalayan salt
- 1 tablespoon coconut oil

Cooking Directions

1. Add all the listed ingredients to your blender (except oil, spices and salt)

2. Blend until smooth
3. Mix in coconut oil, spices, and salt
4. Stir, and enjoy!

Creative Winter Smoothie

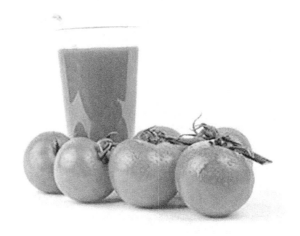

Serving: 2

Prep Time: 5 minutes

<u>Ingredients</u>

- 3 tomatoes, peeled
- 1 celery stalk
- 2 cloves garlic, peeled
- 1-inch ginger, peeled
- 1 cucumber, peeled
- Juice of 1 lemon
- 1 cup alkaline water
- Salt as needed
- Pepper as needed
- Pinch of turmeric
- Olive oil/avocado oil

Cooking Directions

1. Add tomatoes, celery, garlic, cucumber and water to your blender
2. Blend well until smooth
3. Add lemon juice, salt, and oil
4. Stir
5. Season with pepper, and turmeric
6. Stir
7. Serve chilled and enjoy!

Feisty Mango and Coconut Smoothie

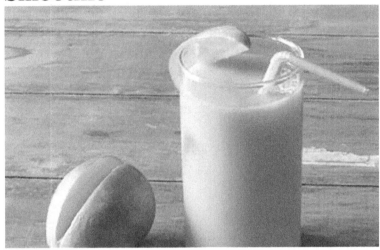

Serving: 2

Prep Time: 5 minutes

Ingredients

- 1 teaspoon spirulina
- 1 cup frozen mango
- 1 cup unsweetened coconut milk
- ½ cup spinach

Cooking Directions
1. Cut mangoes and dice them
2. Add mango, a cup of unsweetened coconut milk, a teaspoon of Spirulina and spinach to your blender
3. Blend on low to medium until smooth
4. Check the texture and serve chilled!

Mexican Chocolate Stand-Off

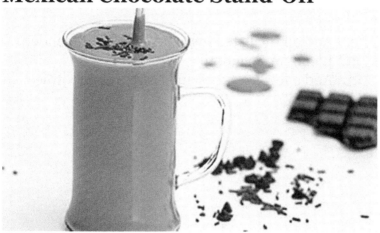

Serving: 2

Prep Time: 5 minutes

<u>Ingredients</u>

- 2 bananas
- 1 tablespoon hemp seeds
- 1 bag frozen blueberries
- ½ teaspoon liquid stevia
- Pure water
- 2 teaspoons raw chocolate
- 1 teaspoon raw carob powder
- ½ teaspoon green powder
- ½ teaspoon cinnamon powder
- Pinch of cayenne pepper

Cooking Directions

1. Add all the listed ingredients to your blender
2. Blend until smooth
3. Add a few ice cubes and serve the smoothie
4. Enjoy!

The Awesome Cleanser

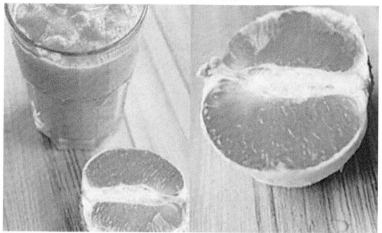

Serving: 2

Prep Time: 5 minutes

Ingredients

- 2 grapefruits, juiced
- 2 lemons, juiced
- Half cup alkaline water/filtered water
- 2 tablespoons olive oil
- 2 cucumbers, peeled
- 1 avocado, peeled and pitted
- 2 cloves fresh garlic
- 1-inch ginger
- Pinch of Himalayan salt
- Pinch of cayenne pepper

Cooking Directions

1. Add cucumber, ginger, avocado, grapefruit, and lemon to your blender
2. Blend until smooth
3. Add alkaline water, spices, and oil
4. Stir well and serve chilled
5. Enjoy!

Gentle Tropical Papaya Smoothie

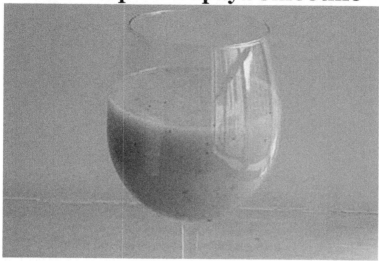

Serving: 2

Prep Time: 5 minutes

Ingredients

- 1 papaya, cut into chunks
- 1 cup fat free plain yogurt
- ½ cup pineapple chunks
- ½ cup crushed ice
- 1 teaspoon coconut extract
- 1 teaspoon flaxseed

Cooking Directions

1. Add the listed ingredients to your blender and blend until smooth
2. Serve chilled!

Kale and Apple Smoothie

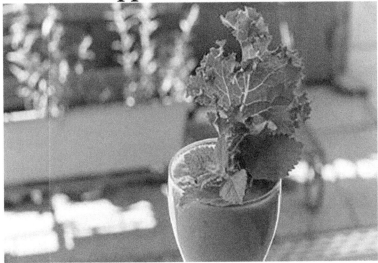

Serving: 2

Prep Time: 5 minutes

Ingredients

- ¾ of a kale, chopped, ribs and stem removed
- 1 small stalk celery, chopped
- ½ a banana
- ½ cup apple juice
- 1 tablespoon lemon juice

Cooking Directions

1. Add the listed ingredients to your blender and blend until smooth
2. Serve chilled!

Mango and Lime Generous Smoothie

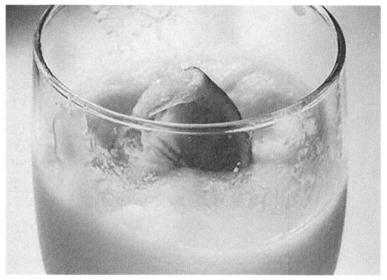

Serving: 2

Prep Time: 5 minutes

Ingredients

- 2 tablespoon lime juice
- 2 cups spinach, chopped and stemmed
- 1 and ½ cups frozen mango, cubed
- 1 cup green grapes

Cooking Directions

1. Add the listed ingredients to your blender and blend until smooth
2. Serve chilled!

The Pear and Chocolate Catastrophe

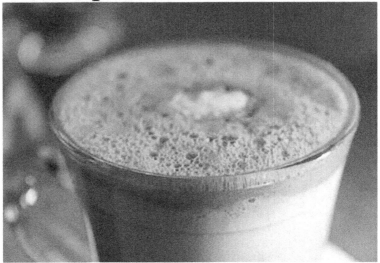

Serving: 2

Prep Time: 5 minutes

Ingredients

- 1 banana (freckled skin)
- 2-3 pears
- 2 tablespoons hulled hemp seeds
- 1 bag frozen raspberries
- 2 and ½ cups coconut water
- 1 teaspoon raw chocolate
- Small bunch arugula lettuce leaves
- Liquid Stevia

Cooking Directions

1. Add all the listed ingredients to your blender
2. Blend until smooth
3. Add a few ice cubes and serve the smoothie
4. Enjoy!

Blackberry and Apple Smoothie

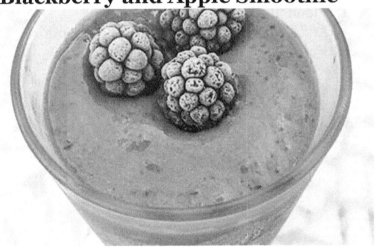

Serving: 2

Prep Time: 5 minutes

Ingredients

- 2 cups frozen blackberries
- ½ cup apple cider
- 1 apple, cubed
- 2/3 cup non-fat lemon yogurt

Cooking Directions

1. Add the listed ingredients to your blender and blend until smooth
2. Serve chilled!

The Mean Green Smoothie

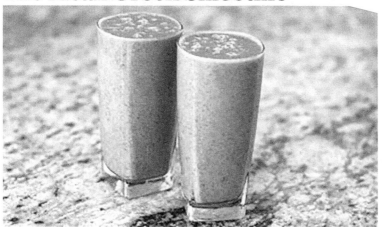

Serving: 2

Prep Time: 5 minutes

Ingredients

- 1 avocado
- 1 handful spinach, chopped
- Cucumber, 2 inch slices, peeled
- 1 lime, chopped
- Handful of grapes, chopped
- 5 dates, stoned and chopped
- 1 cup apple juice (fresh)

Cooking Directions

1. Add all the listed ingredients to your blender
2. Blend until smooth
3. Add a few ice cubes and serve the smoothie
4. Enjoy!

Mint Flavored Pear Smoothie

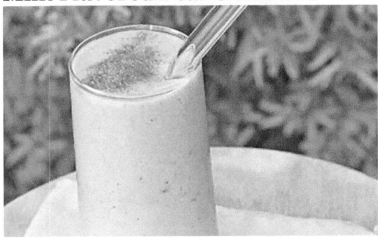

Serving: 2

Prep Time: 5 minutes

Ingredients

- ¼ honey dew
- 2 green pears, ripe
- ½ an apple, juiced
- 1 cup ice cubes
- ½ cup fresh mint leaves

Cooking Directions

1. Add the listed ingredients to your blender and blend until smooth
2. Serve chilled!

Chilled Watermelon Smoothie

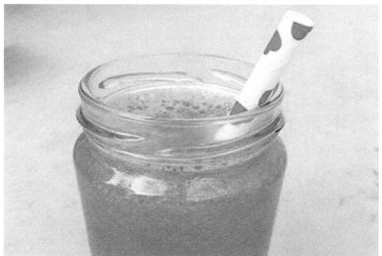

Serving: 2

Prep Time: 5 minutes

Ingredients

- 1 cup watermelon chunks
- ½ cup coconut water
- 1 and ½ teaspoon lime juice
- 4 mint leaves
- 4 ice cubes

Cooking Directions

1. Add the listed ingredients to your blender and blend until smooth
2. Serve chilled!

Banana Ginger Medley

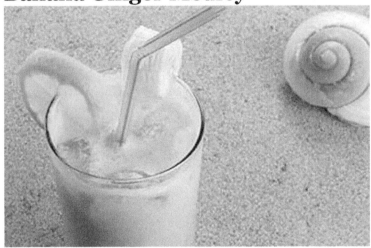

Serving: 2

Prep Time: 5 minutes

Ingredients

- 1 banana, sliced
- ¾ cup vanilla yogurt
- 1 tablespoon honey
- ½ teaspoon ginger, grated

Cooking Directions

1. Add the listed ingredients to your blender and blend until smooth
2. Serve chilled!

Banana and Almond Flax Glass

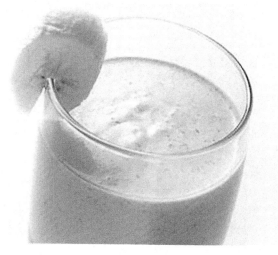

Serving: 2

Prep Time: 5 minutes

Ingredients

- 1 ripe frozen banana, diced
- 2/3 cup unsweetened almond milk
- 1/3 cup fat free plain Greek Yogurt
- 1 and ½ tablespoons almond butter
- 1 tablespoon flax seed meal
- 1 teaspoon honey
- 2-3 drops almond extract

Cooking Directions

1. Add the listed ingredients to your blender and blend until smooth
2. Serve chilled!

Sensational Strawberry Medley

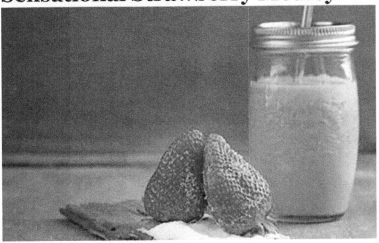

Serving: 2

Prep Time: 5 minutes

Ingredients

- 1-2 handful baby greens
- 3 medium kale leaves
- 5-8 mint leaves
- 1-inch piece of ginger, peeled
- 1 avocado
- 1 cup strawberries
- 6-8 ounces coconut water + 6-8 ounces of filtered water
- Fresh juice of one lime
- 1-2 teaspoon olive oil

Cooking Directions

1. Add all the listed ingredients to your blender

2. Blend until smooth
3. Add a few ice cubes and serve the smoothie
4. Enjoy!

Mango's Gone Haywire

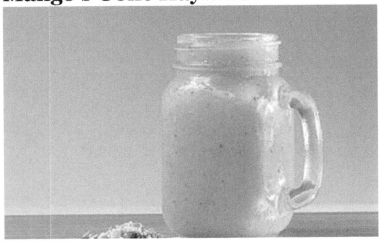

Serving: 2

Prep Time: 5 minutes

Ingredients

- 1 mango, diced
- 2 bananas, diced
- 1-2 oranges, quartered
- Dash of lemon juice
- 1 tablespoon hemp seed
- ¼ teaspoon green powder
- Coconut water (as needed)

Cooking Directions

1. Add orange quarters in your blender first, blend
2. Add the remaining ingredients and blend until smooth
3. Add more coconut water to adjust the thickness
4. Serve chilled!

Unexpectedly Awesome Orange Smoothie

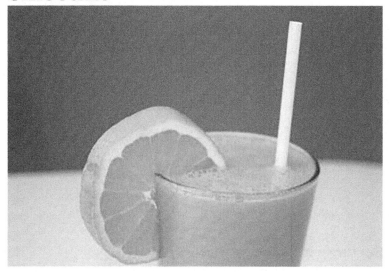

Serving: 2

Prep Time: 5 minutes

Ingredients

- 1 orange, peeled
- ¼ cup fat-free yogurt
- 2 tablespoons frozen orange juice concentrate
- ¼ teaspoon vanilla extract
- 4 ice cubes

Cooking Directions

1. Add the listed ingredients to your blender and blend until smooth
2. Serve chilled!

Minty Cherry Smoothie

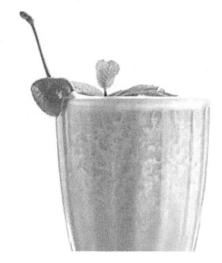

Serving: 2

Prep Time: 5 minutes

Ingredients

- ¾ cup cherries
- 1 teaspoon mint
- ½ cup almond milk
- ½ cup kale
- ½ teaspoon fresh vanilla

Cooking Directions

- Wash and cut cherries
- Take the pits out
- Add cherries to your blender
- Pour almond milk

- Wash the mint and put two sprigs in your blender
- Separate the leaves of kale from stems
- Put kale in your blender
- Press vanilla bean and cut lengthwise with a knife
- Scoop out your desired amount of vanilla and add to your blender
- Blend until smooth
- Serve chilled and enjoy!

A Very Berry (And Green) Smoothie

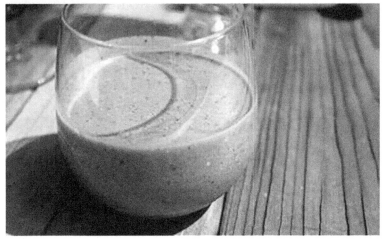

Serving: 2

Prep Time: 5 minutes

Ingredients

- 1 cup spinach leaves
- ½ cup frozen blueberries
- 1 ripe banana
- ½ cup milk
- 2 tablespoon old fashioned oats
- ½ tablespoon stevia

Cooking Directions

1. Add the listed ingredients to your blender and blend until smooth
2. Serve chilled!

Authentic Ginger and Berry Smoothie

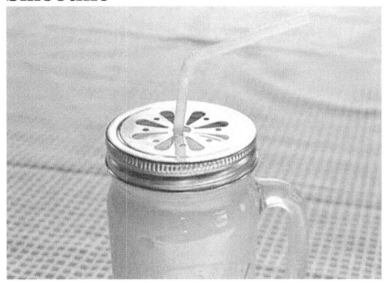

Serving: 2

Prep Time: 5 minutes

Ingredients

- 2 cups blackberries
- 2 cups unsweetened almond milk
- 1 -2 packs of stevia
- 1 piece of 1 inch fresh ginger, peeled and roughly chopped
- 2 cups crushed ice

How To
1. Add the listed ingredients to a blender and blend the whole mixture until smooth
2. Serve chilled and enjoy!

A Glassful of Kale And Spinach

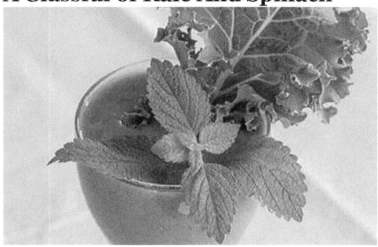

Serving: 2

Prep Time: 5 minutes

Ingredients

- Handful of kale
- Handful of spinach
- 2 broccoli heads
- 1 tomato
- Handful of lettuce
- 1 avocado, cubed
- 1 cucumber, cubed
- Juice of ½ lemon
- Pineapple juice as needed

Cooking Directions

1. Add all the listed ingredients to your blender
2. Blend until smooth

3. Add a few ice cubes and serve the smoothie
4. Enjoy!

Green Tea, Turmeric, And Mango Smoothie

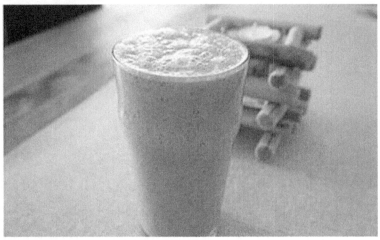

Serving: 2

Prep Time: 5 minutes

Ingredients

- 2 cups mango, cubed
- 2 teaspoons turmeric powder
- 2 tablespoons Green Tea powder
- 2 cups almond milk
- 2 tablespoons honey
- 1 cup crushed ice

How To

1. Add the listed ingredients to a blender and blend the whole mixture until smooth
2. Serve chilled and enjoy!

The Great Anti-Oxidant Glass

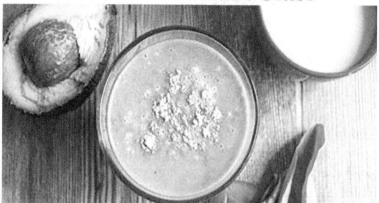

Serving: 2

Prep Time: 5 minutes

Ingredients

- 1 whole ripe avocado
- 4 cups organic baby spinach leaves
- 1 cup filtered water
- Juice of 1 lemon
- 1 English cucumber, chopped
- 3 stems fresh parsley
- 5 stems fresh mint
- 1 inch piece fresh ginger
- 2 large ice cubes

Cooking Directions
1. Add all the listed ingredients to your blender
2. Blend until smooth
3. Add a few ice cubes and serve the smoothie
4. Enjoy!

Conclusion

I would like to thank you for purchasing the book and taking the time for going through it as well. I do hope that this book has been helpful and you found the information contained in the recipes useful! Keep in mind that you are not only limited to the recipes provided in this book! Just go ahead and keep on exploring until you create your very own Smoothie magnum opus!

Stay healthy and stay safe!

Made in the USA
Coppell, TX
17 December 2020

45789113R00056